CLINICAL TRIALS
NARRATIVE

SIDHARTH ANANTHANARAYAN

Clinical Trials Narrative

Place of Publication - India

ISBN - 978-93-5701-468-7

Copyright © 2022 Sidharth Ananthanarayan

Disclaimer

I have made every effort to ensure that the information in this book is accurate in regard to the Clinical Trials, but I do not warranty the details since they can change due to the dynamic nature of the process.

Preface

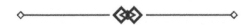

The idea of Clinical Trials Narrative stuck in my mind when I was job hunting and eager to get into Clinical Trial Management. Though I was interested in the end-to-end process, there was minimal information available in one place that I could go over and understand quickly. This book aims to tell the story of Clinical Trials and, most importantly, how can someone interested in working for clinical trials fit into this puzzle. Clinical Trials Narrative provides insights into the overall process of the clinical trials, history around regulations, and career paths in clinical research. With this book, I hope that an aspiring clinical trial professional can walk into the interview with basic knowledge of the overall process and speak the clinical trial language.

Dedication

I dedicate this book to my mother – Lalitha, my sister - Sindhu, and my grandparents – Krishna Iyer and Sudha Krishna Iyer.

I also dedicate this book to my friends Sirish Raghunath and Madhukesh Murthy, with whom I share many memories from my undergraduate days.

Special thanks to all my close friends and acquaintances who constantly support and encourage me in my adventures.

Significant Contributors

Dr. Jithendra Kini Bailur – Dr. Bailur, a Clinical Translational Scientist in a leading pharmaceutical company, contributed significantly to this book with his knowledge of clinical trials. He actively brainstormed and provided information regarding Clinical Trials to help readers understand the narrative.

Varuni M Ankolekar – Varuni, a Data Analyst in a leading Clinical Research Organization, provided valuable input from her experience in Clinical Data Management. She has contributed significantly to the Data Management portions that will help many aspiring clinical trial professionals.

Thanks to Pavitra Kamath, Roxanne Kight, Dr. Sabine Rech, Deepthi Devaraj, Akash Ashok, and Ankitha Verrma for their ideas and inputs.

Table of Contents

Glossary

Acronym	Expansion	Description
ADaM	Analysis Data Model	Specification with significant standards for Analyzing clinical trial datasets
AE/SAE	Adverse Event/Serious Adverse Event	An incident that occurred in a patient that was not expected to happen
CAPA	Corrective Action and Preventive Action	CAPA is the steps taken to address a quality incident and eliminate the root cause to avoid future issues
COV	Close-Out Visit	A final visit to close the sites after the study related activities are completed
CPM	Clinical Project Manager	Acts as a Liaison between the cross functional teams for managing the Clinical Trial
CRA	Clinical Research Associate	Acts as a liaison for assigned Sites. Plays a critical role in reviewing the site-related activities in a clinical trial

CRF	Case Report Forms	A form that sites will use to obtain patient data while participating in the clinical trial
CRO	Contract Research Organization	An organization that provides service to a pharmaceutical company to conduct a clinical trial or other related activities
CSR	Clinical Study Report	Report with detailed information about the outcomes and methods incorporated in a study
CTA	Clinical Trial Agreement	An agreement outlining contractual terms between two site and CRO/Sponsor in a clinical trial
CTM	Clinical Trial Manager	Responsible for managing and overseeing clinical trials and guiding Clinical Research Associates and Clinical Trial Associates
DBL	Database Lock	A Milestone for Clinical Database, no further changes will be allowed from the time of Database Lock
DCGI	Drugs Controller General of India	Health Regulatory authority of India - in charge of evaluating the medicinal products in India

DM	Data Management	Team or Department responsible for overseeing the study data management
DMP	Data Management Plan	Plan outlines the details of managing the patient data entered in the EDC
EDC	Electronic Database	Electronic Database that stores and records clinical data
EMA	European Medical Agency	Regulatory Authority of European Union – in charge of evaluating the medicinal products in the EU
FDA	Food and Drug Administration	Regulatory Authority of the United States of America – in charge of evaluating medicinal products in the US
HIPAA	Health Insurance Portability and Accountability Act	Law outlining the guidelines for flow of patient information
IB	Investigator Brochure	A detailed compilation of information related to the investigational product provided by the sponsor to principal investigators
ICF	Informed Consent Form	Used to record the patient's consent to participate in a clinical trial

ICH-GCP	International Conference on Harmonization-Good Clinical Practice	Guidelines established by International Conference on Harmonization for Good Clinical Practice
IMV	Interim Monitoring Visit	Multiple periodic site visits to review the study progress and documentation at sites
IP	Investigational Product	Drug Products that will be tested in clinical trials to treat an indication
IPM	Investigational Product Manual	Provides details regarding the investigational product, its properties, formulation, and non-clinical study details
IRB	Institutional Review Board	Group of people who the FDA designates to review and approve clinical trials
IRT/IWRS/CTMS	Interactive Response Technology/Interactive Web Response Systems/Clinical Trial Management System	An electronic system used in a study to standardize and conduct the clinical trial
MHLW	Ministry of Health, Labor and Welfare of Japan	Regulatory Authority of Japan– in charge of evaluating medicinal products in Japan
MHRA	Medicines and Healthcare products Regulatory Agency	Regulatory Authority of the UK– in charge of evaluating medicinal products in the UK

MoH – RF	Ministry of Health of the Russian Federation	Regulatory Authority of Russia – in charge of evaluating medicinal products in Russia
NMPA	National Medical Products Administration	Regulatory Authority of China – in charge of evaluating medicinal products in China
PI	Principle Investigator	A physician who is the main lead in conducting a clinical trial at the site
PK	Pharmacokinetics	Helps in determining the fate of the investigational product in the living organisms
PD	Pharmacodynamics	It is the study of drug effect on the living organisms
QA	Quality Assurance	Team or Department overseeing the study to ensure compliance of ICH/GCP guidelines
RACI	Responsibility, Accountable, Consulted and Informed	Table or document with a list of activities with Responsibility Assignment
SAV	Site Activation Visit	Visit conducted to Activate the site that allows them to screen patients

SAP	Statistical Analysis Plan	Plan outlining the statistical methods that will be used for the analysis of the study data
SDTM	Study Data Tabulation Model	Specification for developing tables with human study data
SDV	Source Data Verification	Process of verifying the source document with clinical trial information that is entered in the EDC
SFQ	Site Feasibility Questionnaire	A questionnaire developed to reach out to sites and gather their responses on capabilities and patient population
SIV	Site Invitation Visit	Visit conducted to initiate the site and provide necessary trainings to conduct a clinical trial
SME	Subject Matter Expert	A person with immense knowledge about the subject
SSV/SQV/PSSV	Site Selection Visit/Site Qualification Visit/ Preliminary Site Selection Visit	Site visit to understand the site's capability to conduct clinical trials

TMF	Trial Master File	Central file to store and archive clinical trial documents
UAT	User Acceptance Testing	Testing conducted by end users of the EDC to confirm if the software meets the design specification

Chapter One
Overview of Clinical Trails

Living organisms have a history of millions of years of evolution. Human beings are considered the most evolved organisms in this epic history. As established by the legendary biologist Charles Darwin in his Theory of Evolution, the fittest survive and continue to evolve. During evolution, our body encounters several illnesses, and our immune system must put up its best fight to stop the infection.

Our immune system cannot always be at its best and requires external support from medications. These natural or synthesized medications boost our immune system and give us strength to limit the infection's spread across the body. Providing medicine is not as simple as it sounds; it involves several years of research and understanding.

The synthesized compound is analyzed to understand its attributes and tested to understand its efficacy against infection. The successful compound will then be tested on smaller animals with similar conditions to understand if the same results are recurring. If the compound is

1

successful, it will be tested on humans to confirm that the previous outcomes are accurate and that the compound can successfully limit the infection and boost our immune system.

Testing on humans has always been challenging; several lives were lost due to inaccurate testing practices. There are several grim incidents in humanity's history, but some stand out. The first incident occurred in 1937, Elixir Sulfanilamide was used to treat patients with streptococci infections, and it had shown better results in treating patients in powdered and solid forms. The company developed Elixir Sulfanilamide in a liquid state using Diethylene glycol due to the demand reported by the sales team. The scientists tested Elixir Sulfanilamide only for its flavor and appearance but not toxicity. The consumption of Elixir Sulfanilamide in liquid resulted in the death of more than 100 people. Though the product tasted better and was easy to consume, it was poisonous because of Diethylene glycol. The death of more than 100 people led to the 1938 Federal Food, Drug, and Cosmetic Act; the new law mandated approval by the FDA of any new drug products manufactured and sold for human consumption. It also required the companies to include their drug label with the direction of use and side effects.

The second incident was the Thalidomide tragedy in 1960. In the late 1950s, Thalidomide was sold to treat morning sickness or anxiety (Loue, S, Sajatovic M 2004). During pregnancy, women suffered morning sickness and started to consume Thalidomide. Initially, it was considered safe for pregnant women, but it caused congenital disabilities in several babies born during that period. A total of 10,000 infants were affected, of which 40% died at the time of birth, and the remaining 60% survived with significant health issues (Miller MT, 1991). This incident led to the Drug Amendments Act of 1962; the law required manufacturing companies to list the side effects on their drug label and stop marketing cheap generic products as breakthrough drugs (Meadows, 2006).

The third incident was the Tuskegee Experiment conducted between 1932 and 1972. In this experiment, there were 600 participants - 399 patients had Syphilis, and 201 patients were healthy. The patients received free medical exams, meals, and burial insurance, but the consent of the study participants was not solicited. In 1943, penicillin treated all syphilis patients except study participants. In 1972, an article was published regarding discrimination against the study participants; an Advisory board was appointed to review the study. Based on the discovery of the advisory board, the study was terminated immediately, and the patients started to receive standard-of-care treatment. This incident led to the mandatory involvement of the IRBs to review clinical trials and ensure fair practice and no active discrimination amongst the study participants (Heller. J, 2017).

Along with these three critical regulations, several other important laws and regulations were implemented worldwide to support pharmaceutical companies in identifying the compounds and curing patients with ailing conditions. These regulations also assist in executing clinical trials and obtaining safety and efficacy data. The COVID-19 pandemic has changed lives drastically, but it also taught everyone the importance of testing the vaccine by conducting clinical trials (*also referred to as a study*). Many developed countries conducted clinical trials with many patients participating in them. Though the vaccine was made available to people in a short period, it is not the same in regular times. A clinical trial generally takes several years; it's a long-term, investment-heavy project. The sponsor conducts pre-clinical experiments and clinical trials from Phase I to Phase IV. During these phases, the IP goes through human trials to test its safety and efficacy profile.

In the Pre-Clinical Phase, the IP is tested on animals to understand its safety and efficacy. Different modalities (small molecule, antibody-drug conjugates, cell therapy) are tested during pre-clinical testing. The animals receive different doses of IP to understand their safety and toxicity profile.

In Phase I, a new investigational drug application is submitted to the regulatory authority based on the outcome of Pre-Clinical trials. A full Protocol will be developed and updated based on the regulatory approval of the IND. During Phase I, the IP will be tested on 20 to 100 healthy volunteers or patients with the disease to understand its safety and efficacy at various dosing levels. The efficient dose level identified will be used to test on a larger group of subjects in Phase II.

In Phase II, several hundred patients with disease/ condition will be enrolled in a clinical trial to understand the IP's efficacy and potential side effects. The dose identified in the Phase I study will be used in Phase II. Certain Phase II clinical trials will include a comparison between the control arm and treatment arm to evaluate the efficacy of IP against a placebo/control. The patients will be randomized to the Placebo/Control or Treatment arm and receive a specific amount of IP during the study. The data is analyzed to confirm the efficacy of IP against the placebo/control group after all the patients have completed their visits.

In Phase III, to determine Efficacy, Safety Profile, and Adverse Events (side effects) over a more extended period, 300-3000 patients with the disease will be enrolled in the study. The number of subjects enrolled in a study will depend on the clinical trial indication and statistical power. The Phase III clinical trial is pivotal, and the data readout is essential for the drug product's approval. In clinical trials for rare indications, the number of subjects will be low since the number of patients with the prevailing condition would be less, and the regulatory agencies provide a fast-track pathway to treat these rare indications (Commissioner, 2018).

In Phase IV, the study will primarily focus on patients treated with the newly approved product; the main objective would be to understand any potential side effects that might occur in patients after being treated with the IP. Phase IV study is also known as the Post-Market study.

Clinical Trials are also categorized as therapeutic and non-therapeutic trials:

In a **Therapeutic Trial,** the tested IP will likely benefit the subject, whereas the **Non-therapeutic Trial's** objective is to gain information regarding the product or indication. Non-therapeutic Trials can also include Digital Therapeutic studies to test various software applications or Class I and II medical devices to treat an indication.

The Clinical Trials can also be classified based on study design:

- **Randomized** - In a Randomized Clinical Trial, there are multiple arms, and the patients are triaged to one of the arms to receive treatment. However, most of the study team, subjects, and site team will be unaware if the patient is in the placebo/control group or treatment arm. If any issues might cause unblinding, the unblinded team will handle it.

    o **Single Blind** - Subject is unaware of treatment assignment, i.e., treatment group or a placebo/control group.

    o **Double Blind** - Subject and researcher, are unaware of treatment assignment, i.e., treatment group or a placebo/control group.

- **Open Labeled** - In Open Label Clinical Trial, the IP is used to treat the subjects, and the Subject and Investigator are aware of IP-related information (Anuj, 2016).

Reflection Questions:

1) How many patients might get enrolled in a pivotal study?

2) Is Informed Consent mandatory for participating in a clinical trial?

3) In a Phase-II clinical trial, what study design is followed in this study if a subject and researcher are unaware of the assigned treatment group?

4) What is blinding?

Space for jotting down your thoughts

Space for jotting down your thoughts

Chapter Two
Stakeholders

Clinical trials have several pieces in the puzzle, and it takes immense resources and work hours to complete. Primary resources are the key stakeholders who play distinctive roles and contribute to clinical trial conduct.

Stakeholders in Clinical Trials are:

- **Subject/Patient** - The subject/patient is a key stakeholder in any clinical trial since their consented participation is the crux of the process. They agree to allow a sponsor to test their IP with the hope that it could help them cure the illness.

- **Principal Investigator (PI)** - PI is a physician who will conduct a clinical trial per the GCP guidelines and try to treat their patient with IP to treat the disease. They are responsible for the activities associated with a clinical trial at their site.

- **Sponsor** - A Sponsor is a biotech company with a drug product developed in-house or licensed by an academic institute or another biotech company and wants to test it to treat a specific illness.

- **Contract Research Organizations (CRO)** - CROs are service organizations with extensive resources to execute clinical trials. They offer functional services or End-to-end solutions to execute clinical trials. They have the required workforce to conduct a clinical trial based on the designed Protocol and Regulatory guidelines.

- **Clinical Site** - Clinical sites are clinics, hospitals, or institutions used for conducting clinical trials. Clinical sites recruit volunteer patients for a clinical trial and treat them on study per protocol and GCP guidelines. The number of sites in a clinical trial will depend on the required number of subjects and countries where a study is planned. Other factors, such as startup timelines, costs, capabilities, medical equipment availability, logistics, and trained site staff to perform study procedures, will be considered depending on the site selected for the study.

- **Institutional Review Board (IRB)** - Review boards consist of representatives from various backgrounds that form an independent committee to review clinical trial protocol. They also review Adverse Events reported by sites to assess the impact of IP on patients. There are two types of IRB - Central IRB and Local IRB. The Central IRB is a centralized review board contracted by the Sponsor or CRO for reviewing the study and participating sites. Institutional IRBs are called The Local IRB.

- **Regulatory agencies** - Regulatory agencies will be involved in a clinical trial from the beginning till the end of a clinical trial. Each country will have its regulatory agencies to oversee clinical trial compliance to ICH-GCP and country-specific guidelines. Some important agencies are US - FDA, EU - EMA, UK - MHRA, Japan - MHLW, China - NMPA, India - DCGI, and Russia - RMH.

- **Site Management Organization (SMO)** - SMOs are site service providers; they provide administrative support to PIs. The SMOs act as a point of contact for their sites and handle activities related to IRB submissions, site feasibility, contract negotiation, and patient recruitment.

- **Central Labs** - Central Labs are laboratories with standardized and specialized capabilities to perform various laboratory tests. The site will ship the biological samples of the patients participating in a clinical trial to Central Labs for performing tests per

Protocol.

- **Language Translation Service Provider** - Language Translation Service vendors are critical for global studies. The approved translation vendors will translate study documents for Regulatory Submission and patient-facing documents to assist patients in understanding the study details.

- **Bioanalytical Service Provider** - Bioanalytical services include analysis of Pharmacokinetics (PK), Pharmacodynamics (PD), and Toxicokinetic. Bioanalytics helps understand the behavior of IP on the human body and how the body reacts to the IP.

Reflection Questions:

1) Who is the key stakeholder in a clinical trial?

2) What is the role of a Sponsor in a clinical trial?

3) Which are various regulatory agencies around the world?

4) What is the role of a clinical site in a clinical trial?

Space for jotting down your thoughts

Chapter Three
Study Planning

The following are the stages involved in any clinical trial - Planning, Kick-off, Startup, Conduct, and Close-Out. Various functional teams will be involved in these stages, and they play a pivotal role in executing a clinical trial.

Once the sponsor has identified potential drug candidates, they will initiate the Planning stage for a clinical trial. The preliminary step in the Planning stage would be to identify and earmark necessary resources for the clinical trial. After allocating resources, the sponsor will start identifying stakeholders to conduct the clinical trial.

- **Identify the Stakeholders** - The sponsor would be the primary stakeholder who owns the IP and wants to bring it to the patients who need it. To make this possible, the sponsor's study Team will identify and contract with a CRO capable of conducting clinical trials. Based on the contract, the assigned team at the CRO will support and carry out a site feasibility process to identify the clinical sites and investigators with the target subject population and infrastructure to execute a clinical trial. The CRO's CPM will request resources from Clinical Operations, Data Management, Data Sciences, Medical Writing, Regulatory, Safety and Pharmacovigilance, Supply Chain, and Quality Team. The functional heads will allocate the resources necessary for a clinical trial based on the request of the CPM. The Sponsor's CTM/CPM and CPM at CRO will work on identifying the required vendors for conducting a clinical trial; in several instances, the CRO will propose potential vendors while bidding for the clinical trial contract with the sponsor.

- **Define Objectives** - Cross-functional teams of the Sponsor and CRO will work together to define the objectives of clinical trials based on the Protocol; this process is critical to understanding the expected outcome and helps develop a roadmap to achieve the objective.

- **Protocol Development** - A Protocol is developed for each clinical trial and is a guide with a step-by-step process to conduct a clinical trial. Several stakeholders, such as Clinical Biostatisticians, Regulatory SMEs, Physicians, Clinical Translation SMEs, etc., provide their inputs during protocol development. The Protocol includes the following essential topics:

- o Introduction - It outlines the indication, the IP details, and the studied population. It also includes descriptions of potential risks and benefits for the patient, along with previous clinical trial data (Clinical Trial Protocol Development, 2017).

- o Protocol Synopsis - Protocol Synopsis summarizes a Clinical Trial protocol. It includes - Title, Study Objectives, Patient Population, Study Design, Schedule of Assessments, Inclusion and Exclusion Criteria, Endpoints, and Statistical Analysis. The summarized information helps understand the overview of a study, and it is helpful for stakeholders to review any critical information about the study (Clinical Trial Protocol Development, 2017).

- o Study Objectives - The study objectives include a clinical trial's primary and secondary objectives. The objectives will highlight hypotheses and the purpose of conducting the clinical trial (Clinical Trial Protocol

19

Development, 2017).

o Study Endpoints - The endpoints are mostly quantitative measurements of the objectives. The endpoints are always well defined to help determine accurate outcomes of a clinical trial (Clinical Trial Protocol Development, 2017).

o Statistical Considerations - Statistical Considerations are the most critical aspect of a Protocol. Biostatisticians determine statistical power based on the study objectives. Power determination helps define the statistical methods to measure the endpoints and determine the number of patients that need to be enrolled and treated in a study to achieve the desired outcome (Clinical Trial Protocol Development, 2017).

o Inclusion and Exclusion or I/E criteria - It is a set of characteristics the subject needs to pass during screening for study enrollment. These criteria are related to a patient's condition, such as blood pressure, sugar levels, pregnancy, and medications (Clinical Trial Protocol Development, 2017).

o Study Assessments - Study Assessments are the tests conducted during a subject's visits while participating in a clinical trial. These tests could be subjective or bioanalytical. The subject answers specific questions in a subjective test, and the site staff records them. The site staff will draw blood for bioanalytical tests and ship it to Central Labs or Bioanalytical Service Labs (Clinical Trial Protocol Development, 2017).

o Data Handling - The details of platforms and processes are included in the Data Handling section for site staff to enter, manage, and archive patient information. This section also explains the steps to protect patients' privacy and comply with the HIPAA guidelines (Clinical Trial Protocol Development, 2017).

• **Understand the Budget Allocation** - The budget is a predetermined amount of funds for each functional group executing a clinical trial. The Sponsor and CRO will negotiate and agree upon the contract terms and budget; the terms are listed in the contract and signed. After executing the contract between the Sponsor and CRO, the project management team will

21

review the budget breakdown to understand cost allocation. A Budget Breakdown review is crucial since it provides an opportunity to identify potential over-promised and undervalued activities. Identifying such activities will help in anticipating a potential risk of cost overrun in the future. The sponsor will pay CRO for any responsibilities of managing vendors or clinical sites.

- **Contract Vendors** – The vital step is to contract Vendors while the Budget breakdown is thoroughly analyzed. Critical vendors in a clinical trial would be Electronic Data Capture (EDC), Trial Master File (TMF), Safety Database, Interactive Response Technology (IRT) Systems, and Drug Depot.

  - The EDC - It is used in a clinical trial to track the patient visit details, test results, IP dispensing, randomization, and other critical information; the leading EDC systems are IBM and Medidata Rave, owned by IBM and Dassault Systems, respectively.

  - The TMF - Each clinical trial will have thousands of documents that record the activities conducted, and archiving these documents is necessary to tell a clinical trial's story. Leading TMF software such as Veeva Systems, TransPerfect, and Oracle are used to archive clinical trial documents.

o Safety Database - Its purpose is to track Adverse Events (AE), Serious Adverse Events (SAE), and concomitant medication details in a clinical trial. It helps track all safety incidents in a clinical trial - the most commonly used Safety Database is Argus.

o IRT Systems - The IRT systems are mainly used to streamline data exchange between Clinical Site, Sponsor, and CRO. Using a centralized platform to track the patient status will help the Sponsor and CRO manage the patients and help Supply Chain to ship the IP to sites as per the timeline for dosing. There are several leading IRT vendors, and they are selected depending on the needs of a clinical trial.

o Central Lab - The Sponsor or CRO will contract the Central Labs to perform standardized tests per Protocol. The sites will ship patient samples to Central Lab, and the lab will perform various tests and upload the results to a central location for analysis.

- Drug Depot - Drug Depots are necessary to ship the IP and ancillary supplies to clinical sites. For clinical trials conducted in multiple countries, the Drug Depot vendor is essential for importing the IP into the country and shipping it to clinical sites. The drug depots will use Cryo Shippers to ship the IP to sites; it contains Liquid Nitrogen which helps maintain the IP'S storage temperature while in transit.

- *Please note - In most cases, the Quality Assurance (QA) team at the CRO will already have qualified vendors, but if there is a need for a new vendor, they will have to be qualified by the QA team. After identifying the vendor, the QA team will schedule a vendor audit; during this audit, the QA team will review their relevant SOPs to understand their operating practices. The QA team will record the audit findings in their compliance audit report. The vendor will not be qualified until the issues are resolved and meet the qualification criteria. The QA team will issue a certificate to use the vendor for clinical trials. The QA team will review qualified vendors periodically to ensure their compliance.*

- **Develop a Project Management Plan** - Project Plan/ Timeline/Work Breakdown Structure is a detailed list of tasks that lead to Milestones planned in a Clinical Trial. A Project Plan would consist of details of tasks, their start and end dates, the number of hours required to complete a task, and resources assigned to the task. This level of detail helps track the task status and resource utilization. The project plan also helps forecast potential delays caused by various factors; this will help the project management team develop Risk and Issue mitigation strategies. Microsoft Project and Smart sheets are preferred tools for project planning.

- **Develop Materials for Kick-off Meeting** - The kick-off meeting is an essential milestone in any Clinical Trial. It is a meeting that brings together various stakeholders who will be part of a clinical trial. It is necessary to develop material that will give detailed insights into the study, overall communication structure, and responsibilities of various teams. During this meeting, the cross-functional teams review the Protocol, study timelines, plans, and EDC build status. The critical study plans will be discussed and finalized during the kick-off meeting. One of the essential plans would be the communication plan; the

Communication Plan will act as a guide to understanding the communication lines between the stakeholders involved in a clinical trial. Since several teams are involved in a clinical trial, the project management team is responsible for maintaining the communication lines and ensuring the information transfer to respective stakeholders. The project management team will maintain a live document containing all the stakeholders' contact details.

- **Schedule Kick-off Meeting** - The CPM will schedule a Kick-off meeting after reviewing necessary information, identifying stakeholders, contracting vendors, and drafting the plans/materials for the kick-off meeting. The team would start the planning stage with a target kick-off meeting date in mind. As the date comes closer, it is the responsibility of the project management team to decide the venue to accommodate necessary travel plans.

Reflection questions:

1) What are the critical sections of a Protocol?

2) Why is a Budget review critical in a clinical trial?

3) Who are the key vendors in a clinical trial?

4) What is the use of a project plan?

5) When does the Kick-off meeting occur?

Space for jotting down your thoughts

Chapter Four
Kick-off Meeting

The kick-off meeting could typically be two days with multiple sessions on the agenda. CPM would lead the first session to introduce the Sponsor to all stakeholders attending the Kick-off meeting. The following sessions will be on various topics listed on the agenda for the Kick-off meeting. Amongst those topics, the two key topics would be a discussion with the Data Management (DM) team regarding EDC Go-Live and Vendor discussions. These two are critical aspects since they play a significant role in Clinical Trial Conduct.

- During the EDC Go-Live discussion - The sponsor and DM team will review the study details, roles, and responsibilities of the Sponsor and CRO for EDC Go-Live, unique CRFs, and Train the team to use the EDC.

- During the vendor discussion - The contractual terms, timelines for service delivery, and roles and responsibilities of the vendors participating in the clinical trial are discussed with the Sponsor. The crucial vendors would be for the IRT system, Drug Depot to import the IP to other countries, central lab for performing lab tests, and Courier vendor to ship the ancillary supplies or IP. The project management team and the Sponsor will determine if a Central IRB will be necessary for the Clinical Trial.

The other important aspect covered in a Kick-off meeting is the discussion of plans with the Sponsor. It serves as a guidance document during the clinical trial Conduct. During the Kick-off meeting, the project management team and the Sponsor might discuss the following plans:

- Communication Plan - The Communication Plan outlines the details of various stakeholders who will be part of the study and highlights their responsibilities. The plan includes stakeholders' contact details and their preferred communication path.

- Monitoring Plan - The Monitoring Plan outlines details of Site Monitoring responsibilities. The plan guides a CRA to schedule necessary Monitoring Visits at the site and complete the required activities while on Site.

- Data Management Plan (DMP) - DMP outlines the details of managing the patient data entered in the EDC. It also includes guidance for the DM team to review data entered in EBC.

- eTMF Plan - eTMF Plan outlines the platform used as eTMF and the operating instruction to upload documents to the eTMF. The plan also includes Nomenclature and codes to classify the documents while uploading.

- Vendor Management Plan - Vendor Management Plan includes detailed instructions on managing vendor interactions. The plan provides instructions to escalate vendor issues during the clinical trial Conduct.

- Other plans - Medical Monitoring Plan, Data Validation Plan, and Statistical Analysis Plan are other key plans discussed briefly during the Kick-off meeting.

Along with the plans, discussion of timelines is also critical during the Kick-Off meeting. The CPM will share a Project Plan with detailed timelines to achieve set milestones in the Clinical Trial. The team will also review any milestones that might be at risk and discuss risk mitigation strategies. Reviewing timelines/Project plans during the kick-off meeting will allow all the stakeholders to highlight any of their concerns.

During the kick-off meeting, the CRO team might utilize the opportunity to demonstrate the Clinical Trial Management System, Site Payment Platform, and IRT platform to the Sponsor. It helps the Sponsor understand the tools and monitor study progress, patient enrollment, query resolution status, and AEs.

RACI is an acronym for _Responsibility Accountable Consulted and Informed_. RACI discussion could be another important topic on the agenda; RACI is a matrix with a list of activities and stakeholders responsible for completing the activity. RACI helps in developing a structure and clarifying responsibilities in a clinical trial. _Table 1 is an example of the RACI Chart used in the Industry._

	Sponsor	**CRO**	**Vendor**
Regulatory Approval	R, A	C, I	I
Communication Plan	C	R, A	I
Platform Development	C	I	R, A

Table 1: Example of a RACI Chart

Other topics, such as Regulatory Approval timelines and Scientific discussion around the Protocol, could be covered during the Kick-off meeting. Completion of the Kick-off meeting is a significant milestone achievement in a study.

Investigator Meeting - Investigator meetings will help review the Protocol with investigators participating in the study. The Sponsor's chief medical officer or Chief Investigator of the clinical trial will usually lead the meeting. Investigator meetings allow physicians to discuss the study design, mechanism of action of the IP, and potential benefits for patients.

Reflection Questions:

1) Who are the key participants in a kick-off meeting?

2) What are the plans that might be discussed in a Kick-off meeting?

3) What is the use of a RACI?

Space for jotting down your thoughts

Space for jotting down your thoughts

Chapter Five
Study Startup

Preliminary study activities performed during the Study Startup phase are critical to the successful Conduct of a Clinical Trial irrespective of the study outcome/efficacy results.

During Startup Phase, the following activities are accomplished:

- **Regulatory approvals** - Regulatory approval is the official approval from the Regulatory Authority to conduct a clinical trial. The Sponsor's Regulatory Team or CRO's Regulatory Team, on behalf of the Sponsor, submits the regulatory dossier/packet to seek approval for conducting a Clinical Trial in the country of interest. Each regulatory authority has a specific timeline to review the application and provide approval. Each country has different requirements that the sponsor or CRO must comply with while submitting the dossier/packet. The dossier/packet will include a New Drug application, clinical trial protocol, drug product import license,

Investigator CV, and other documents specific to the country. During the review, the Regulatory agency will go over the Protocol to understand the risks and benefits for the patients. In addition, they might also review the experience of the Chief Investigator in conducting studies related to the indication. There could be feedback to update the Protocol in case the committee believes there is a higher risk that can impact the patients. The regulatory approvals are on the Critical Path in a project plan due to the potential delay if a study is not approved; this emphasizes the need for appropriate planning for regulatory submission to avoid delays in receiving the approval. Once the approval is received, the Regulatory Team will update the study details on clinicaltrials.gov and submit an annual study report to the regulatory authority.

- **Protocol Review** - The CRO and Sponsor team might review the Protocol before starting any study-related activities to incorporate any potential feedback from PIs participating in the study.

- **Create Study-related Documents** - The Medical Writing team will work closely with various functional teams to develop several critical documents used in a Clinical Trial. Some of the important ones are:

- *Informed Consent Form (ICF)* - The ICF is used to obtain a Subject/Patient's consent to participate in the Clinical Trial. The ICF contains detailed information on potential risks and benefits of participating in the study; it is the PI's responsibility to review the ICF with the Subject or their parents/relatives if the Subject is under 18 years of age and cannot consent to be part of the study. The ICF also includes the patient's responsibilities while participating in the study. If the Subject consents to a study but feels uncomfortable proceeding further at a later stage, they can withdraw their consent and discontinue the study.

- *Investigator Brochure (IB)* - The IB is a study document developed by the Sponsor and distributed to Investigators who will be part of the Clinical Trial. The IB has information regarding IP's physical, chemical and pharmaceutical properties. It also includes a summary of any non-clinical study data and guidance to the Investigator.

- o *Investigational Product Manual (IPM)* - The IPM is a document developed by the Sponsor; it provides instructions to Pharmacists and Site staff for handling the IP while preparing it for dosing the subject. It also includes instructions for storing the active IP. Along with IP handling instructions, the IPM might contain instructions regarding requesting ancillary supplies for the Clinical Trial.

- **Site Feasibility** - Site Feasibility is a process where the CPM/Site Feasibility team reaches out to potential clinical sites and investigators with experience in treating patients who are under consideration for the study. The site and investigator details available in several databases are used in site feasibility. The team will develop a Site Feasibility Questionnaire (SFQ) based on the study Protocol and send it to potential investigators along with the blinded Protocol Synopsis and Confidentiality Agreement. The Confidentiality Agreement is provided to an investigator to sign off and return to the CRO or sponsor. The objective of the confidentiality agreement is to agree to legal terms of not disclosing details of the Protocol and study design. The Sponsor or CRO will share the unblinded Protocol once the Confidentiality Agreement is signed. Some investigators review blinded Protocol and respond to SFQ, whereas some prefer to review full Protocol and provide responses to the SFQ. The CPM compiles and analyzes the responses to recommend the best sites with the necessary infrastructure and patient population. The CPM will forward the responses from sites to the sponsor for their review and approval of recommended sites for the Site Selection Visit.

- **Site Selection Visit (SSV) or Site Qualification Visit (SQV)** - Once the sponsor approves the Site for SSV, a CRA gets assigned to the site. The project management team will request the Site Staff to provide the CV and Medical License of the Investigator for their records. The CRA will contact the Investigator or his team member and schedule a time for SSV or SQV. The SSV/SQV could range from 4 hours to a full working day; during the visit, CRA will review the checklist they have put together after reviewing the Protocol and schedule of events in the study. The SSV/SQV provides site staff and PI an opportunity to understand and discuss the study. The CRA will also assess site infrastructure, pharmacy, staffing, and equipment available for the study. After completing the site visit, the CRA will report the findings to the Clinical Operations and CPM teams. The report will be reviewed and discussed with the Sponsor; if the report is positive, the Sponsor might approve the site, and if it is negative, the Sponsor might not approve it. The CRA will send a follow-up letter to the site with the study team's detailed response and decision.

- **Database Go-Live** - It is a critical milestone in a study, and the following steps will complete Go-Live and ensure the build of EDC as per the specifications:

  - **Development and testing of eCRF form:**

    - The DM Team will create a study within the architecture of the EDC development tool, followed by the creation of non - production environments and sites

    - Designer/Programmer identifies eCRFs required for the project, adds them to the study created within the EDC development tool, and modifies the eCRFs specific for the trial

- The DM Team will recognize the mappings, dynamic fields or forms, data fields for IRT, and data points as per Coding dictionaries. The visit schedule will be designed based on the schedule of events in the Protocol, and dynamics are programmed accordingly

- The programmer and DM team test the eCRFs once the programming is complete

- The DM team will discuss the eCRF design with the Sponsor and incorporate any recommended changes

- The Sponsor will approve eCRFs after finalization by the DM Team

- **Development of IRT:**

  - IRT plan is created and discussed with the study team and IRT vendor

  - IRT development meetings are set up, and the IRT is designed as per the specifications by the sponsor or DM team

  - The DM team performs the end-to-end testing per specifications

- The sponsor approves IRT after testing is complete

- The IRT is moved to production by the vendor

o **Medical Coding setup:**

- It is necessary to set up coding of medical terms to have a unique medical term for a particular ailment. Standard dictionaries are available for coding AEs, Concomitant Medications, and Medical History (e.g., MedDRA, WHODrug). Coding can be automated or performed manually

o **Targeted Source Data Verification (tSDV):**

- The clinical operations lead determines critical SDV requirements

- After recognizing data points for SDV, programming is completed and tested to ensure the required fields have an SDV check box enabled the in the EDC

o **Development of Edit Check Specification:**

- Edit check specification is a document with rules written to get a notification or query when there is a discrepancy in data entry. It includes edit checks, dynamics, derivations, and email alerts on critical data points

- Edit checks are drafted based on the eCRFs fields in a study. Edit check specifications are reviewed and approved by the sponsor DM team

  o **Performing User Acceptance Testing (UAT):**

    - The programming gets initiated based on the UAT Plan once the edit check specification is approved. The DM team writes test scripts as per specifications

    - The programmer completes programming and notifies the team to start UAT

    - The DM team performs testing based on the test scripts; the authors of test scripts will not perform the testing for their cases

      i. For Local lab eCRFs, normal lab ranges for each test are entered in the lab module and linked to the respective lab forms. The DM team will perform UAT by referring to the lab ranges module

ii. If there are any comments, the tester communicates them to the programmer or DM team. The DM Team or programmer will make the updates based on observations

iii. Upon fixing all the issues, the EDC would be ready for Go-live

- The EDC is moved to production after all approval documents are received

- **Other documents created during the setup phase:** Along with DMP and Edit check specifications, the DM team will create the following documents during the setup phase:

  o eCRF completion guidelines - Includes detailed information regarding CRF pages in the EDC. It instructs site staff to enter the data in EDC and guides the DM team in data cleaning activities

  o Coding guidelines - Provides instructions on how to perform coding for AEs, Medical History, Concomitant Medication, and other medical terms

- o <u>SAE reconciliation plan</u> - Provides guidelines to ensure all SAEs and AESIs (Adverse Event of Special Interest) recorded in the EDC and safety database are consistent

- o <u>Protocol Deviation guidelines</u> - Describes the process of managing deviations from the Protocol

- o <u>eCRF Specification</u> - Describes the details regarding eCRF design, fields present in the eCRF and acceptable format, and control type for each field

- o <u>Annotated CRF</u> - Describes the annotation or mapping of fields present in the eCRF to corresponding fields in the datasets

- **Budgeting** - The budgeting in the startup phase is for paying the clinical sites participating in a study. Based on the type of study and required tests in Protocol, Sponsor's team conducts market research to understand the potential costs of performing these tests in a clinical site. Based on the outcome of market research, Sponsor will create a budget template. The CPM will provide the budget template to selected sites post-SSV or SQV.

Reflection Questions:

1) Which study-related documents will be developed during the Startup stage of a Clinical Trial?

2) Why is Site Feasibility an essential step in a clinical trial?

3) What is the objective of SSV or SQV in a clinical trial?

Space for jotting down your thoughts

Space for jotting down your thoughts

Chapter Six
Study Conduct

The shortlisted sites are informed, and the Clinical Trial Conduct stage begins. The Sponsor or CRO will provide a copy of the budget and Clinical Trial Agreement (CTA) to a Selected Site for their review. The Site will review the budget and give a counteroffer with administrative cost details for conducting a clinical trial. The Sponsor will review and approve the counteroffer budget or negotiate with the site to accept a middle ground if necessary. The Site will review the CTA terms and respond to the Sponsor with any proposed changes; if the sponsor agrees with the proposed changes, they will accept and execute the CTA. If proposed changes by the site are not entirely acceptable, the Sponsor will try to negotiate terms and complete the CTA. *Please note - that there will be instances when a site or sponsor might not accept the budget or proposed terms in the CTA or both; at that time, the Site will not participate in the clinical trial.*

After CTA execution, the important step for a site would be to initiate the IRB review process. As explained earlier, the

IRB is a review board of members from various backgrounds; they review the Protocol, approve a clinical trial, and periodically review the study to ensure compliance with GCP/ICH guidelines. The IRB committee can also request sponsors to alter some parts of the study design if they have any concerns. Institutional sites usually have their own IRB committees that review Clinical Trial Protocols; however, the sites can work with IRB engaged by the Sponsor or CRO. The Sponsor/CRO will contract with a centralized IRB to support all clinical sites participating in their study. The Sponsor/CRO will provide site and PI details to the IRB; sites will then have to provide all required documents to the IRB for their review and approval to conduct the study. The Sponsor/CRO and each site must apply for an annual IRB review until the study is closed. The Sponsor will pay for costs incurred for the IRB review.

After the CTA finalization and IRB approval, the following activities are conducted at each site:

- **Shipping of Investigational Product and Ancillary Supplies** - IP and Ancillary Supplies will be shipped to the Site by the Sponsor/CRO. Ancillary supplies include screening kits, dosing kits, and blood draw kits. It will be replenished if necessary, depending on the expiry or requirement for sites to screen and enroll more patients. Depending on the dosing schedule IP (or placebo control if a Clinical Trial is placebo-controlled) gets shipped to the Site. The Supply Chain team will coordinate shipment from Drug Depot and ensure timely delivery of the IP for the patient's dosing. There will be instances when the patient might have to reschedule for dosing; in such instances, the IP will either be stored or destroyed based on the guidelines in IP Manual. If the site is in a different country, an import license is necessary to import the IP into that country and ship it to the site. Another critical component is customs clearance when IP is shipped from the manufacturing site to a Drug Depot in a different country. It is a critical path and should be planned well in advance to avoid delays in customs.

- **Site Initiation Visit (SIV)** - Once the CTA is signed off, the next step would be to initiate the site. CRA will discuss with the PI to schedule an SIV and send out a confirmation letter with a confirmed date and time. During SIV, the CRA will train site staff & PI on the schedule of events, protocol assessments, data entry process in the EDC, and IP handling. The Sponsor and CRO will create training material and demonstration videos that the CRA will use to complete trainings during the SIV. The trainings are critical, and the CRA must document the completion of these trainings in the SIV Training Log to ensure compliance.

- Usually, sites get activated during SIV, but if there are any pending activities, Site Activation is conducted later. After the SIV and Site Activation, the DM Team enables patient screening for the Site on EDC and IRT. After the patient signs the informed consent, they enter the Screening phase; then, the site staff will perform Screening assessments to verify if the patient meets the study-specific inclusion and exclusion criterion, which helps determines a subject's eligibility to patriciate in a clinical trial. If a patient does not meet the criteria, they would be declared a screen fail.

- **Enrollment Monitoring** - After completing the screening and determining eligibility, the site will randomize the patient. When enrolled in a study, patients will receive an active drug product or placebo/control. The patient goes through the assessments listed in the Protocol. The site staff will enter the assessment results into the EDC. CRA and DM will review test results to ensure data is accurate and there are no discrepancies. *Please note - that the patient has the right to discontinue or withdraw their consent from a clinical trial.*

The first patient being randomized and dozed in the clinical trial marks a milestone called First Patient First Visit (FPFV); it is tracked in Project Plan to calculate the number of days taken to achieve the FPFV milestone. The CPM will use similar milestones to track 25%, 50%, 75%, and 100% of patients enrolled in the clinical trial. It is essential to monitor the enrollment to understand potential risks in enrolling patients in the study. The significant risks that usually occur in clinical trials are a higher screen failure rate and patients discontinuing the study due to difficulty following the protocol procedures. Enrollment tracking helps develop risk mitigation strategies to resolve risks and complete the Clinical Trial with the required number of patients. Enrollment monitoring also helps to understand the performance of each site. The CRA and CPM initiate dialogue with the PI to understand the reasons for lower enrollment if the site enrolls fewer patients than estimated during feasibility.

- **Central Lab and Local Lab setup** - Site staff will ship the blood and other biological samples to Local Labs or Central Labs to perform protocol assessments and evaluate the patient's PK and PD values. There are several assays performed to determine the PK and PD values.

  o The Sponsor or CRO usually contracts central labs to perform various tests in a clinical trial. The lab vendor will transfer clinical test data to the Sponsor/CRO based on accepted Data Transfer Specifications. The Sponsor/CRO DM team will reconcile the data and provide it to the Biostatistics team for analysis.

  o Local Labs are usually contracted or located in-house at a clinical site to perform specific assays/tests. The test results data will be entered in the EDC using eCRFs. The CRA will review the data during the IMV.

- **Interim Monitoring Visits (IMV)** - IMV will be conducted periodically for each clinical trial to ensure compliance. CRAs will obtain the availability of site staff and provide a confirmation letter to schedule the IMV. It is primarily on-site, but there are instances when certain IMVs are conducted remotely by securing necessary source data from the site and reviewed online. Each site will maintain an IMV Log with dates, CRA details, and other information to track the visits. During the IMV, CRA will review Source Documents and perform SDV of data entered in EDC CRFs. The SDV is necessary to ensure the data transcribed is accurate based on the clinical trial requirement. If there are any discrepancies, the CRAs will raise queries to the site and seek correction or explanation for the discrepancy. CRA will also support the site and guide them to resolve any active queries raised by the DM team or the CRA themself during their previous visit. CRAs will also review the IP accountability log to ensure no discrepancy in IP dispensation to patients. CRA will also discuss with the PI any potential issues at the site related to the Clinical Trial and communicate them to the Sponsor or CPM for resolution.

- **AE/SAE Reporting** - AE/SAEs are unexpected events during a Clinical Trial. The classification of AEs is in a broad range, but some examples could be high or low blood pressure, frequent headaches, allergic reactions, cough, cold, or fever. SAEs, on the other hand, are incidents that could cause patient hospitalization or lead to death. All AEs and SAEs must be reported using the AE/SAE reporting guidelines and saved in the safety database. Safety Medical Monitor and the Pharmacovigilance team will review the reported AE/SAE to understand if the patient needs to be taken off the study to provide necessary treatment. The Safety and Pharmacovigilance team needs to provide subject safety narratives and evaluate the safety report. In case of any AEs leading to death, hospitalization, congenital anomaly/congenital disabilities, life-threatening, or other medical abnormalities, the Safety and Pharmacovigilance team needs to report it to the regulatory authority and inform other PIs in the study. If necessary, the sponsor will pause the clinical trial until the regulatory authority provides further guidance. Since the advent of Cell and Gene therapy, there have been multiple instances where clinical trials are paused or discontinued due to SAE. The DM & Safety Team frequently reconcile the adverse events to ensure they are consistent and complete.

- o The Safety Team is also responsible for Medical Coding activities; they will review the AEs and ConMeds entered by the site for a patient during the clinical trial Conduct; they will code each AEs and ConMeds using the MedDRA and WHO Drug Dictionary.

- ○ The site coordinator will enter the patient data into the EDC after the patient completes screening. After data entry, the DM team will perform their activities per DMP and other specific plans for the Clinical Trial.

- **Data Management activities** - The following DM activities are performed during the study conduct stage:

  - ○ **Query Management** - The site will be notified via query if there are any discrepancies in the CRF. The query will be closed or re-queried based on the response or update.

  - ○ **External data reconciliation** - The DM team will reconcile lab and imaging data from Central labs with the source documents based on the data transfer agreement. If there are discrepancies in the data entry, queries will be issued to rectify errors.

  - ○ **SAE reconciliation** - The DM team will reconcile SAEs recorded in both safety and clinical databases per the SAE reconciliation plan to ensure data is consistent between the databases.

o **Local lab data review** - The DM Team reviews the protocol assessment results entered by the Local lab and raises queries for any missing, inappropriate, or abnormal results. If the result is abnormal, the query will be to confirm the clinical significance of the entered data.

o **Protocol Deviation review** - Any deviation from the Protocol would be considered critical; The DM Team will review the deviations per the Protocol deviation guidelines document and categorize them as a Major or Minor Protocol Deviation.

o **Data Validation/Dataset review** - The DM Team will review every CRF for its completeness and accuracy.

o **Database Migration** - After a Protocol amendment or due to a sponsor requirement, if there is a need to update the EDC or CRF pages, the programmer will analyze necessary updates and code for changes after obtaining necessary approvals. The tester will then complete the testing and document findings; the Database will be pushed to production and released after all issues get addressed.

o **Data Safety Monitoring Board/ Data Monitoring Committee review** - The committees intermittently review the data in production to analyze the safety and efficacy of the investigational product. It will help determine trends and decide on the continuation or discontinuation of the Clinical Trial accordingly. In most Clinical Trials, the DM Team will perform an Interim Database Lock based on the timelines set by the Sponsor, the data is cleaned based on the data cutoff date, and the data will be soft locked or frozen.

o **Freezing the CRF** - After reviewing and addressing all discrepancies, CRF is soft-locked/frozen to restrict further changes. However, if necessary, it can be unfrozen to update any queries.

o **Locking the CRF** - CRF can be hard-locked only after it is soft-locked or frozen, after which the Investigator can review and sign the CRFs.

- **Study Data Tabulation Model (SDTM) Coding** - After Clinical Startup, the SAS Programmers get assigned to the Clinical Trial. The SAS Programmer will create the specifications for SDTMs based on the Protocol and begin coding for the SDTMs; After coding the SDTMs, another SAS programmer will perform the validation of SDTMs. Outcomes of SDTM validation will be discussed with the SAS programmer to address any issues or discrepancies. SAS Programmers will complete the Programming and Validation cycle until all issues get resolved. After the final run, the SDTMs get transferred to the Biostatistician. All identified issues will be documented in a report and signed off by the verifying SAS programmer.

- **Analysis Data Model (ADaM) Coding** - Along with SDTM, another important activity would be developing ADaM. During SDTM coding, the SAS Programming team will define the scope and specifications of ADaM. Once the SDTM outputs are received, the SAS programmer will begin coding to transform the SDTM outputs to ADaM. After completing coding, the Validation SAS Programmer will develop and validate the code created by the development SAS Programmer. All the issues identified will be documented and discussed with the Development SAS Programmer to resolve them. After completing the coding, another SAS Programmer will validate the code to fix the issues. The Development and Validation cycle will continue until there are no issues in the code. A Final Run will be conducted for SDTM and ADaM to ensure the codes can run without human intervention; the Programming and Validation details get documented and archived in the TMF.

- **Statistical Analysis Plan (SAP)** - Another important responsibility of the Data Science team would be to develop an (SAP) for analyzing the Clinical Trial Data. SAP holds the key to telling the story of how the drug was safe and effective for patients. The experienced Biostatistician will develop the Statistical Analysis Plan. The plan will include the details of study objectives, study arms, analysis methods to calculate the drug product efficacy, statistical models to calculate the power, Tables, Listings, and Figures, and any analysis supporting the objectives. The SAP will also include details of study design, randomization, blinding, inclusion and exclusion criteria, and study assessments. The SAP consists of considerations for the patient population for the analysis (*i.e., ITT - Intent* *to Treat, Per Protocol Population, and Safety Population*), any subgroups or covariates in the clinical trial, and missing data in the clinical trial.

The SAP will provide details of methods used to analyze the Efficacy and Safety Endpoints; this is an integral part of SAP since the chosen method helps the Physicians and Safety Monitoring Committee determine if the drug was successful. The SAP will also contain guidelines to summarize the Safety Data Points such as AE, SAE, ConMeds, Laboratory Evaluations, pregnancies during a clinical trial, etc. The SAP will include details of any Interim Analysis conducted during the Clinical Trial. The SAP incorporates statistical models suitable to determine the power. If the CRO is developing the SAP, the Sponsor team will review the plan and provide inputs to ensure important details are incorporated.

During SAP development, the programmers will create Tables, Listings, and Figures that will be the statistical analysis output. After defining the scope in SAP, Development Programmers will develop mock TLFs with dummy data. The Validation Programmer will review mock TLFs to ensure the titles, headers, figures, etc., are accurate and provides the necessary output as expected. The discrepancies are documented and communicated to the Development Programmer. The mock TLFs will be validated to ensure there are no discrepancies. A final TLFs test run will be conducted before the Database is locked and the data transferred for Statistical Analysis.

- **Site Audits** - The QA team can perform site audits depending on the site's performance. The QA team will constantly review deviations reported by the team; if there is a particular site that has many deviations reported, the QA team will audit the site. During the Site Audit, the team will try to understand the root cause of issues and identify potential risks with the site's operating procedures. The QA team will provide an audit report to the Site, Sponsor and CRO; the site will be responsible for addressing any findings during the audit and include the Corrective Actions and Preventive Actions (CAPA) in the Audit response. After the Site addresses identified issues, the QA team will issue a certificate that must be filed in TMF along with the Audit report. Depending on the severity of the findings, the site may be disqualified or not allowed to enroll patients in the clinical trial.

- **TMF Audit** - The internal or external QA Auditor will also conduct frequent TMF audits to ensure the timely archiving of the study-related document. These audits help the sponsor understand gaps and documentation practices in the TMF. The Auditor will provide an audit report, and the report will include major and minor findings. Depending on the severity, the functional teams will address the findings with CAPA. Cross-functional teams must provide an audit response after addressing all the findings.

Reflection Questions:

1) Which critical tasks should be completed before scheduling an SIV?

2) What are the topics covered by CRA in an SIV?

3) Why is an IMV conducted in a clinical trial?

4) What are the critical DM activities in the Conduct stage of a clinical trial?

5) Why is an SAP developed in a clinical trial?

Space for jotting down your thoughts

Chapter Seven
Study Close-Out

Once the Last Patient in the Clinical Trial completes their treatment, the Last Patient Last Visit (LPLV) milestone is considered complete. Achieving the LPLV milestone is a reminder to the Study team to verify any pending source data, resolve all open queries, and complete any pending activities in the Database. It paves the way for the critical step - Database lock.

- **Database Lock** - As soon as LPLV is complete, the DM Team will perform the final cleaning of data present in the CRF.

  - For Database Lock, the DM team performs the following activities:

    - Query management

    - Ensure all the coding activities are complete

    - Ensure there are no missing pages or visits

    - Final external data reconciliation

    - Final SAE reconciliation

- Final Protocol deviation review

- Data validation/Dataset review

- DM reviews of the eCRFs

- Freezing/locking the eCRFs

- Signing off all the main pages on EDC along with DMP and other DM-related documents

  o After a final review of reconciliation and query closure, eCRF forms are locked, and the Investigator signs them. Upon database lock, EDC users will have read-only access to the EDC. The Biostatistician will receive the Dataset extracts from the DM team for statistical analysis.

- **Statistical Analysis** - Statistical Analysis is a process where all the Clinical Trial data is analyzed based on the SAP to understand the safety and efficacy of a drug product by measuring the outcomes. The Statistical Analysis results will be presented using the ICH E9 Statistical Principles for Clinical Trials and CONSORT statement.

- **Close-Out Visits (COV)** - Once the Database is locked, CRAs will prepare to initiate the Close-Out Visit process. CRAs will schedule a COV on site to ensure all the IP gets accounted for or destroyed based on the protocols at the site. CRAs will help the project management team to receive any pending documentation from the site that is critical for the study. The CRA will also provide an official close-out letter releasing the site from any responsibilities. However, the site agrees to maintain the study records for a specific period and agrees to cooperate with the Auditor if the regulatory agency audits the site for drug product approval. After COV, the site will inform the IRB about the study closure of their sites.

- **TMF finalization** - The Sponsor might contract with external service providers to audit the TMF for reviewing documents archived in the TMF. The audit helps understand the TMF status compared to the Essential Document List. This opportunity helps fill any gaps with the original document, updated document, or Note to File. If the CRO is responsible for the TMF, they will address all the gaps and transfer the TMF to Sponsor. The Sponsor will utilize documents for the CSR and maintain the TMF for regulatory audit while submitting for marketing authorization of the drug product. TMF gets finalized after auditing all documents archived in the TMF.

- **Study close-out** - During the study close-out, the CRO confirms that all the sites and contracts have been closed. The sponsor or CRO will finalize the payments to vendors contracted in the study and close their agreements. The study EDC will be decommissioned, and the DM team will transfer all the data to the Sponsor for archiving per the guidelines. The CRO or Sponsor will inform the IRB regarding Clinical Trial closure and update the outcomes on clinicaltrials.gov. The Sponsor will notify the regulatory agencies regarding the study close-out and outcomes with the help of a CSR.

- **Clinical Study Report (CSR)** - The CSR is an extensive report with all essential details about the clinical trial. It includes approximately 14 appendices; each appendix contains information regarding the study, essential study documents, information about the investigators, their CVs, Medical licenses, regulatory approvals obtained to conduct the clinical trial, IP manufacturing information, EDC snapshots, TLFs, and statistical analysis. The Medical Writing team incorporates all the necessary appendices based on the clinical trial, and the sponsor will review the appendices. The Medical Writing team will incorporate the comments from the sponsor into the draft. After finalizing the appendices, Medical Writer will incorporate essential documents, TLFs, and Study Outcomes into the CSR. The Biostatistics team will review and approve the information incorporated into the CSR, and the CSR is sent to the Sponsor for their final review and approval. Once the Sponsor approves, the CSR will be finalized and published. This step concludes the study activities.

Reflection Questions:

1) What are the critical tasks performed before locking the Database?

2) What are the responsibilities of a CRA in a COV?

3) What is a CSR, and what is the purpose of developing a CSR?

Space for jotting down your thoughts

Space for jotting down your thoughts

Chapter Eight
Career Paths in Clinical Research

The clinical trial Conduct requires several resources with various skill sets. Every stakeholder has a distinct role to play in completing a clinical trial. Various hard skills are necessary to conduct a clinical trial, but interpersonal skills also play an equally important role. Mastering hard and interpersonal skills can help an individual make the best career in clinical trial management.

Note: Key Activities are a general description of duties; they will vary with each organization and each clinical trial.

Stakeholder	Role	Key Activities
Sponsor/ CRO	Sr. Clinical Trial Manager/ Clinical Trial Manager	Responsible for planning, initiating, and conducting clinical trials and responsible for the functional team involved in the clinical trial

Sponsor/ CRO	Clinical Research Associate	Responsible for liaising with the site and communicating with the PI regarding study progress and helping them address any questions in the study Conduct
Sponsor/ CRO	Clinical Trial Specialist/Clinical Trial Associate	Responsible for project status tracking, minutes taking, communicating with internal stakeholders, and collecting documents.
Sponsor/ CRO	Sr. Clinical Project Manager/ Clinical Project Manager	Responsible for Liaising with the stakeholders and providing updates. Manage functional groups and oversee the budgetary approvals.
Sponsor/ CRO	Clinical Project Lead	Responsible for Liaising with the stakeholders and gathering updates. Responsible for managing certain vendors in a Clinical Trial.

Sponsor/CRO	Clinical Project Associate	Responsible for working with internal teams to gather study updates and maintain trackers. Responsible for document gathering and updating training records for the cross-functional team.
Sponsor/CRO	Sr. Data Manager/Data Manager	Responsible for overseeing the EDC database from Go-Live to Database Lock. Responsible for communicating with the stakeholders and providing necessary updates
Sponsor/CRO	Data Management Lead	Responsible for overseeing the EDC implementation and managing the assigned study team to complete day-to-day activities. Responsible for reports and metrics from the EDC.
Sponsor/CRO	Clinical Data Analyst	Responsible for performing day-to-day data validation and data cleaning activities. Responsible for UAT during the Database Go-live and Migration, Data Reconciliation, and Data Monitoring.

Sponsor/ CRO	Sr. Biostatistician	Responsible for designing statistical methods for clinical data analysis based on the Protocol. Responsible for Liaising with the clinical trial team to plan and execute the SAP
Sponsor/ CRO	Biostatistician	Responsible for developing the SAP for TLF generation. Support the Programming team in report generation for Interim and Final analysis of clinical data.
Sponsor/ CRO	Sr. Statistical Programmer	Responsible for overseeing and supporting coding and testing of the SAS programs for Clinical data analysis. Responsible for managing the team and providing updates to stakeholders. *SAS Certification is required for this role*

Sponsor/ CRO	Statistical Programmer	Responsible for coding, testing, and maintaining SAS programs for Clinical Data analysis. Responsible for programming for TLFs. *SAS Certification is required for this role*
Sponsor/ CRO	Sr. Medical Writer/ Medical Writer Lead	Responsible for leading the development of Clinical documents and working with stakeholders to gather their inputs during the development of these documents. Responsible for managing the medical writing team.
Sponsor/ CRO	Associate Medical Writer	Responsible for creating and editing Clinical Trial documents based on the guidance from Sr. Medical Writer. Responsible for coordinating with functional teams while reviewing documents and updating them based on their inputs.

Sponsor/ CRO	Sr. Regulatory Affairs Manager/ Regulatory Affairs Manager	Responsible for reviewing and supporting the preparation of Regulatory submission packets/dossiers for a Clinical Trial. Provides an update to cross-functional teams regarding submission status.
Sponsor/ CRO	Sr. Regulatory Affairs Associate/ Regulatory Affairs Associate	Responsible for preparing Regulatory submission packets/dossiers for Clinical Trials. Support the cross-functional team in developing documents based on document specifications
Sponsor/ CRO	Sr. Manager Quality Assurance/ Manager Quality Assurance	Responsible for overseeing the compliance during Clinical Trial Conduct. Responsible for supporting the team in addressing any Quality Incidents.
Sponsor/ CRO	Quality Assurance Associate	Responsible for maintaining Quality Assurance documentation, developing reports and metrics of quality incidents and quality audits

Sponsor/ CRO	Vendor QA Manager	Responsible for conducting Qualification Audits of vendors and providing certificates to the team for utilizing their service for the study. Responsible for conducting and maintaining periodic Quality Assurance review
Sponsor/ CRO	Sr. Manager/ Manager Drug Safety and Pharmacovigilance	Responsible for reviewing the AE/SAE reports and providing guidelines based on the inputs from Safety Physician
Sponsor/ CRO	Drug Safety and Pharmacovigilance Associate	Responsible for reviewing safety data and tracking the AE reports provided by the clinical sites
Sponsor/ CRO	Sr. TMF Manager/ TMF Manager	Responsible for liaising with the study team for TMF maintenance. Responsible for setting up the TMF structure and providing access to the study team.

Sponsor/CRO	TMF Administrator	Responsible for managing and reviewing Essential documents and uploading them to TMF. Responsible for overseeing the TMF status.
Sponsor/CRO	TMF Associate	Responsible for reviewing, uploading, and routing the essential documents for the study team's approval.
Sponsor/CRO	Supply Chain Manager	Responsible for forecasting, managing, and coordinating the supply of IP and supplies to the clinical site
Sponsor/CRO	Supply Chain Associate	Responsible for documenting and ordering the supply of IP to sites
CRO/Vendor	Vendor Project Manager	Responsible for managing test orders and providing the results to the Sponsor
CRO/Vendor	Vendor Project Coordinator	Responsible for tracking the test orders, documenting and updating the status of tests to the Sponsor
Site	Principle or Sub Investigator	Responsible for leading a study at a clinical site or institute
Site	Site Manager	Manages the clinical site and oversees clinical trial activities

| Site | Site Coordinator | Responsible for managing day-to-day activities of clinical trial Conduct at the site |
| IRB | IRB Manager | Responsible for coordinating and processing the IRB review applications for various clinical trials |

Space for jotting down your thoughts

References

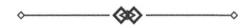

- Anuj, T. (2016, December 24). *Types of clinical research/ trial/studies*. CLINI INDIA. Retrieved August 1, 2022, from http://www.cliniindia.com/hindi/types-of-clinical-researchtrialstudies/

- Clinical Trial Protocol Development, University of California San Francisco, (2017, October 03), Retrieved from https://hub.ucsf.edu/protocol-development

- Commissioner, O. of the. (2018, January 4). *Step 3: Clinical research*. U.S. Food and Drug Administration. Retrieved August 1, 2022, from https://www.fda.gov/patients/drug-development-process/step-3-clinical-research

- Heller, J. (2017, May 10). *AP was there: Black men untreated in tuskegee syphilis study*. AP NEWS. Retrieved August 1, 2022, from https://apnews.com/article/business-science-health-race-and-ethnicity-syphilis-e9dd07eaa4e74052878a68132cd3803a

- Loue S, Sajatovic M (2004). Encyclopedia of Women's Health. Springer Science & Business Media. p. 644.

ISBN 9780306480737.)

- Meadows, M. (2006, February). *Promoting safe and effective drugs for 100 years*. FDA Consumer magazine. Retrieved August 2, 2022, from https://www.fda.gov/files/Promoting-Safe-and-Effective-Drugs-for-100-Years-%28download%29.pdf

- Miller MT (1991). "Thalidomide embryopathy: a model for the study of congenital incomitant horizontal strabismus". Transactions of the American Ophthalmological Society. 89: 623–74. PMC 1298636. PMID 1808819

About the Author

Sidharth Ananthanarayan is a Cell Therapy Operations Specialist at Atara Biotherapeutics. He graduated with a Master's in Biotechnology from San Jose State University, California, and joined the Industry in 2019.

Hailing from a small town near Bengaluru, India. He was inspired by his grandfather's contribution to the welfare of patients and always aimed to contribute to healthcare research to help people with ailing conditions. The inspiration helped him complete his education and start his career in Clinical Trial Management, a significant milestone in his life. This book is a compilation of his learnings about Clinical Trials and career opportunities.